The Definitive Guide to Plant-Based Lunch

Based Lunch

A Complete Collection of Soups, Stews and Meals to Start Your Diet and Boost Your Lunch

Toby Hancock

Table of contents

Spicy Bean Stew

Preparation time: 5 minutes Cooking time: 50 minutes
Servings: 4

Ingredients:

7 ounces cooked black eye beans 14 ounces chopped tomatoes 2 medium carrots, peeled, diced 7 ounces cooked kidney beans 1 leek, diced ½ a chili, chopped 1 teaspoon minced garlic 1/3 teaspoon ground black pepper 2/3 teaspoon salt 1 teaspoon red chili powder 1 lemon, juiced 3 tablespoons white wine 1 tablespoon olive oil 1 2/3 cups vegetable stock

Directions:

Take a large saucepan, place it over medium-high heat, add oil and when hot, add leeks and cook for 8 minutes or until softened. Then add carrots, continue cooking for 4 minutes, stir in chili and garlic, pour in the wine, and continue cooking for 2 minutes. Add tomatoes, stir in lemon juice, pour in the stock and bring the mixture to boil. Switch heat to medium level, simmer for 35 minutes until stew has thickened, then add both beans along with remaining ingredients and cook for 5 minutes until hot. Serve straight away.

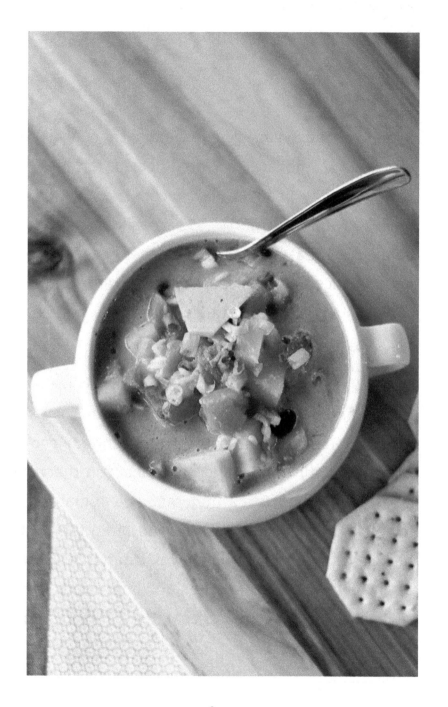

White Bean Stew

Preparation time: 5 minutes Cooking time: 10 hours and 10 minutes Servings: 10

Ingredients:

2 cups chopped spinach 28 ounces diced tomatoes 2 pounds white beans, dried 2 cups chopped chard 2 large carrots, peeled, diced 2 cups chopped kale 3 large celery stalks, diced 1 medium white onion, peeled, diced 1 ½ teaspoon minced garlic 2 tablespoons salt 1 teaspoon dried rosemary ½ teaspoon Ground black pepper, to taste 1 teaspoon dried thyme 1 teaspoon dried oregano 1 bay leaf 10 cups water

Directions:

Switch on the slow cooker, add all the ingredients in it, except for kale, chard, and spinach and stir until combined. Shut the cooker with lid and cook for 10 hours at a low heat setting until thoroughly cooked. When done, stir in kale, chard, and spinach, and cook for 10 minutes until leaves wilt. Serve straight away.

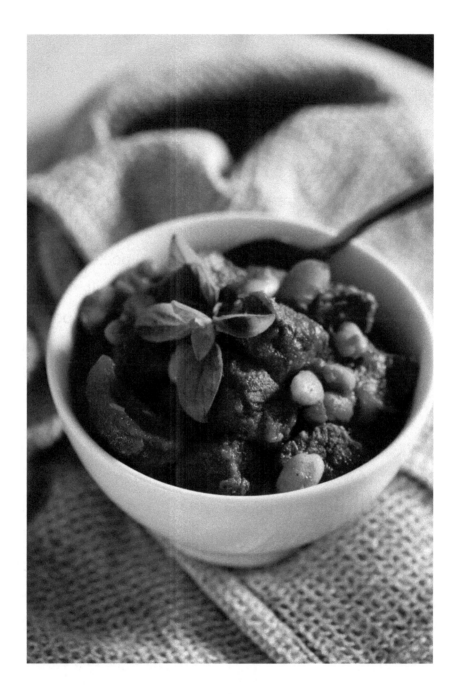

Vegetarian Gumbo

Preparation time: 10 minutes Cooking time: 45 minutes Servings: 4

Ingredients:

1 1/2 cups diced zucchini 16-ounces cooked red beans 4 cups sliced okra 1 1/2 cups diced green pepper 1 1/2 cups chopped white onion 1 1/2 cups diced red bell pepper 8 cremini mushrooms, quartered 1 cup sliced celery 3 teaspoons minced garlic 1 medium tomato, chopped 1 teaspoon red pepper flakes 1 teaspoon dried thyme 3 tablespoons all-purpose flour 1 tablespoon smoked paprika 1 teaspoon dried oregano 1/4 teaspoon nutmeg 1 teaspoon soy sauce 1 1/2 teaspoons liquid smoke 2 tablespoons mustard 1 tablespoon apple cider vinegar 1 tablespoon Worcestershire sauce, vegetarian 1/2 teaspoon hot sauce 3 tablespoons olive oil 4 cups vegetable stock 1/2 cups sliced green onion 4 cups cooked jasmine rice

Directions:

Take a Dutch oven, place it over medium heat, add oil and flour and cook for 5 minutes until fragrant. Switch heat to the medium low level, and continue cooking for 20 minutes until roux becomes dark brown, whisking constantly. Meanwhile, place the tomato in a food processor, add garlic and onion along with remaining ingredients, except for stock, zucchini, celery, mushroom, green and red bell pepper, and pulse for 2 minutes until smooth. Pour the mixture into the pan, return pan over medium-high heat, stir until mixed, and cook for 5 minutes until all the liquid has evaporated. Stir in stock, bring it to simmer, then add remaining vegetables and simmer for 20 minutes until tender. Garnish gumbo with green onions and serve with rice.

Root Vegetable Stew

Preparation time: 10 minutes Cooking time: 8 hours and 10 minutes Servings: 6

Ingredients:

2 cups chopped kale 1 large white onion, peeled, chopped 1 pound parsnips, peeled, chopped 1 pound potatoes, peeled, chopped 2 celery ribs, chopped 1 pound butternut squash, peeled, deseeded, chopped 1 pound carrots, peeled, chopped 3 teaspoons minced garlic 1 pound sweet potatoes, peeled, chopped 1 bay leaf 1 teaspoon ground black pepper 1/2 teaspoon sea salt 1 tablespoon chopped sage 3 cups vegetable broth

Directions:

Switch on the slow cooker, add all the ingredients in it, except for the kale, and stir until mixed. Shut the cooker with lid and cook for 8 hours at a low heat setting until cooked. When done, add kale into the stew, stir until mixed, and cook for 10 minutes until leaves have wilted. Serve straight away

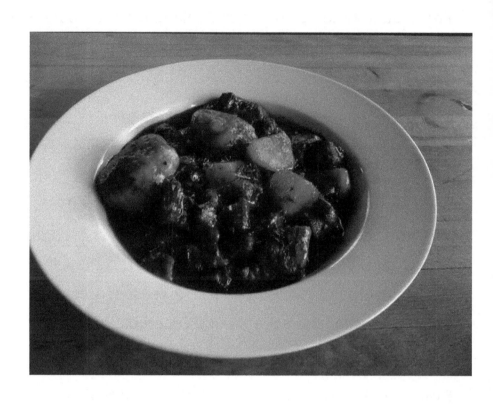

Chopped Kale Power Salad

Preparation time: 10 minutes Cooking time: 40 minutes Servings: 4

Ingredients:

For the Salad: 15 ounces cooked chickpeas 8 cups chopped kale 6 cups diced sweet potatoes 1 large avocado, pitted, diced 1/4 cup chopped red onion 2 teaspoons and 1 tablespoon olive oil, divided 1/4 teaspoon ground black pepper 3/4 teaspoons salt, divided 1/3 cup chopped almonds 1/2 of a large lemon, juiced 1/3 cup dried cranberries

For The Lemon Tahini Dressing: 1/2 cup tahini 1/4 teaspoon salt 1 lemon juiced 6 tablespoons warm water

Directions:

Place diced sweet potatoes on a sheet pan, drizzle with 2 teaspoon oil, season with ¼ teaspoon black pepper and ½ teaspoon salt and bake for 40 minutes at 375 degrees F until roasted, tossing halfway. Meanwhile, place chopped kale in a bowl, drizzle with lemon juice and remaining oil, season with remaining salt, toss until combined, and massage the leaves for 1 minute. Prepare the dressing and for this, place all of its ingredients in a bowl and whisk until combined. Top kale salad with sweet potatoes, drizzle with tahini dressing, and serve.

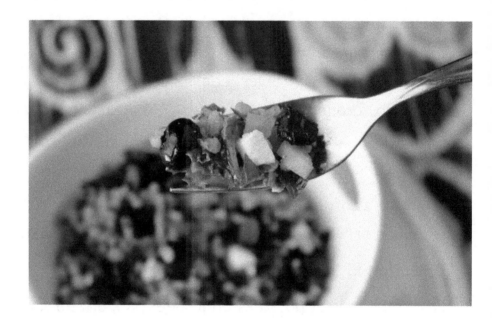

Pear, Pomegranate and Roasted Butternut Squash Salad

Preparation time: 10 minutes Cooking time: 10 minutes Servings: 3

Ingredients:

1 medium butternut squash, peeled, cut into noodles 5 ounces of arugula 1 large pear, spiralized ¾ cup pomegranate seeds 2/3 teaspoon salt 1/3 teaspoon ground black pepper 3/4 cup chopped walnuts For the Vinaigrette: ½ teaspoon minced garlic 1 teaspoon white sesame seeds ¼ teaspoon ground black pepper 1 tablespoon maple syrup 1 tablespoon olive oil 1 tablespoon soy sauce 1 tablespoon sesame oil 2 tablespoons apple cider vinegar

Directions:

Place butternut squash noodles on a baking sheet, spray with oil, season with salt and black pepper and roast for 10 minutes at 400 degrees F until cooked. Meanwhile, prepare the vinaigrette and for this, place all its ingredients in a bowl and whisk until combined. When done, place pear, walnuts, and arugula in a large bowl, then add squash, drizzle with vinaigrette and toss until combined. Serve straight away.

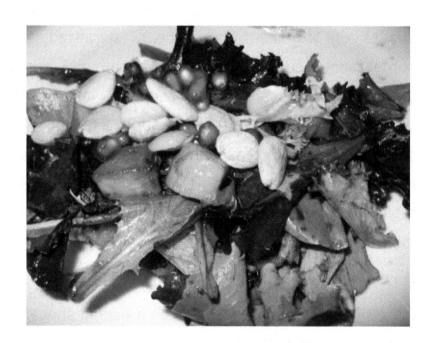

Black Bean Taco Salad

Preparation time: 10 minutes Cooking time: 30 minutes
Servings: 4

Ingredients:

For the Black Beans: 1 1/2 cups cooked black beans
1/2 teaspoon garlic powder 1/2 teaspoon salt 1/2
teaspoon cayenne 1/2 teaspoon smoked paprika 2
teaspoons red chili powder 1 teaspoon cumin 1/4 cup
water

For the Roasted Chickpeas: 1 1/2 cups cooked
chickpeas 1/2 teaspoon salt 1 teaspoon red chili powder
1/4 teaspoon cinnamon 1 teaspoon cumin For the Salad:
1 medium red bell pepper, cored, diced 1 medium head
of green leaf lettuce 1 cup fresh corn kernels 2 chopped
tomatoes 1 avocado, pitted, diced For the Dressing: 1 ½
cup vegan Cumin Ranch Dressing

Directions:

Season chickpeas with salt, cinnamon, chili powder, and cumin, spread them in an even layer on a baking sheet and bake for 30 minutes at 400 degrees F until roasted, stirring halfway. Meanwhile, prepare the black beans and for this, place them on a skillet pan, add remaining ingredients, stir until well mixed and cook for 5 minutes until warmed, set aside until required. Assemble salad and for this, place all its ingredients in a bowl, toss until mixed, then add roasted chickpeas and black beans, drizzle with ranch dressing and serve.

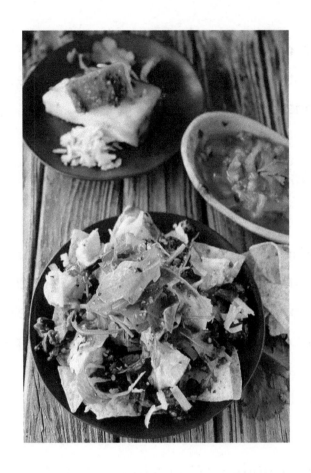

Roasted Vegetable and Quinoa Salad

Preparation time: 10 minutes Cooking time: 25 minutes
Servings: 4

Ingredients:

For the Roasted Vegetables: 1 carrot, peeled, chopped 1 medium sweet potato, peeled, chopped 1 red bell pepper, cored, cubed 1 zucchini, peeled, cubed 1 tablespoon dried mixed herbs 1 red onion, peeled, sliced 1 tablespoon olive oil 1/2 teaspoon salt ¼ teaspoon ground black pepper

For the Quinoa: 1/2 cup frozen peas 1 1/2 cup cooked quinoa 1 cup chopped kale

For the dressing: 1 teaspoon minced garlic 1/4 teaspoon salt 1/4 teaspoon cinnamon 1/2 teaspoon ground cumin 3 tablespoons tahini 1/2 teaspoon brown rice syrup 2 tablespoons olive oil 3 tablespoons lemon juice

Directions:

Place all the vegetables in a large baking dish, season with salt and black pepper, sprinkle with herbs, drizzle with oil, toss until mixed, and then bake them for 25 minutes at 392 degrees F until roasted. Cook the quinoa in a saucepan, add kale and peas in the last three minutes, and when done, let it stand for 10 minutes. Prepare the dressing, and for this, place all of its ingredients in a blender and pulse until smooth. Place everything in a large bowl, drizzle with dressing and toss until mixed. Serve straight away.

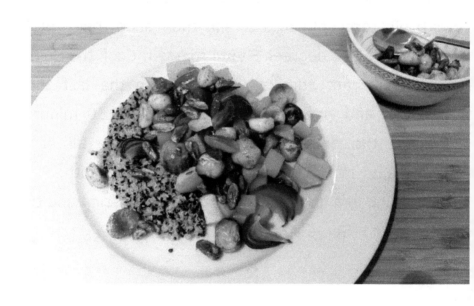

Lentil Fattoush Salad

Preparation time: 10 minutes Cooking time: 7 minutes
Servings: 2

Ingredients:

For the Salad: 1/3 cup green lentils, cooked ¼ small cucumber, chopped 2 stalks of celery, chopped 1 small radish, peeled, sliced 4 cups arugula 1 carrot, chopped ¼ cup dates, chopped 1/3 teaspoon salt 2 teaspoons olive oil 1 pita pocket, whole-wheat, chopped 2 tablespoons toasted sunflower seeds

For the Vinaigrette: 1 tablespoon Dijon mustard 2 tablespoons balsamic vinegar 1 tablespoon maple syrup 2 tablespoons olive oil

Directions:

Place pita pieces on a cookie sheet lined with parchment paper, drizzle with oil, and season with salt, toss until mixed, spread evenly, and bake for 7 minutes at 425 degrees F until golden, and when done, cool them. Meanwhile, prepare the vinaigrette and for this, place all of its ingredients in a bowl and whisk until combined. Add remaining ingredients in a bowl, add cooled pita chips, drizzle with vinaigrette and toss until mixed. Serve straight away.

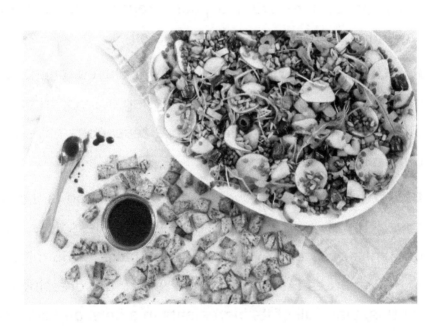

Sweet Potato Salad

Preparation time: 10 minutes Cooking time: 35 minutes
Servings: 4

Ingredients:

2 large sweet potatoes, peeled, 1 1/2 inch cubes 1/3
teaspoon ground black pepper 1/2 teaspoon salt 1/2
teaspoon paprika 1/2 teaspoon oregano 1/2 teaspoon
cayenne pepper 1 tablespoon olive oil

For the Dressing: 1 small bunch of chives, chopped 1
medium shallot, peeled, diced 2 spring onions, trimmed,
diced 1 tablespoon maple syrup 2 teaspoons olive oil 3
tablespoons red wine vinegar

Directions: Spread sweet potato cubes on a baking
sheet, drizzle with oil, season with all the spices, toss
until mixed, spread evenly, and then bake for 35 minutes
at 390 degrees F until roasted. Prepare the dressing and
for this, place all of its ingredients in a bowl and stir until
combined. When sweet potatoes have roasted, let them
cool for 10 minutes, then drizzle with salad dressing and
serve straight away.

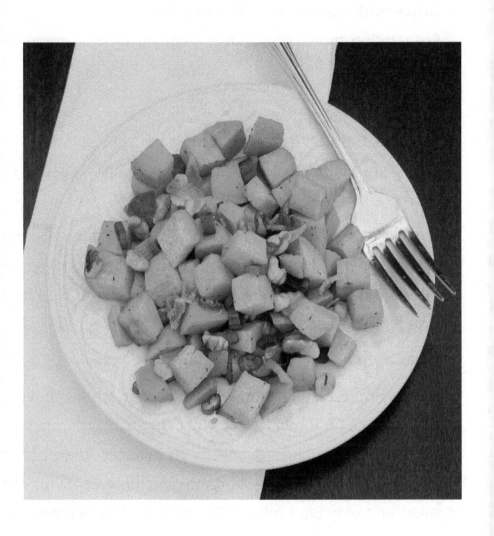

Butternut Squash and Kale Salad

Preparation time: 10 minutes Cooking time: 8 minutes Servings: 4

Ingredients:

For the Salad: 6 cups butternut squash, spiralized 5 cups kale, chopped, steamed 1/3 cup pumpkin seeds 1/2 cup pomegranate seeds

For the Dressing: ½ teaspoon salt ½ teaspoon ground black pepper 1/2 teaspoon cinnamon 1 tablespoon maple syrup 1/2 teaspoon mustard 2 tablespoons apple cider vinegar 3 tablespoons olive oil

Directions:

Place spiralized squash on a baking sheet, toss with olive oil and bake for 8 minutes at 400 degrees F until roasted. When done, let squash cool for 10 minutes, then add it into a large bowl along with remaining ingredients for the salad and toss until mixed. Prepare the dressing and for this, place all of its ingredients in a bowl and stir until combined. Drizzle the dressing over the salad, toss until mixed, and then serve.

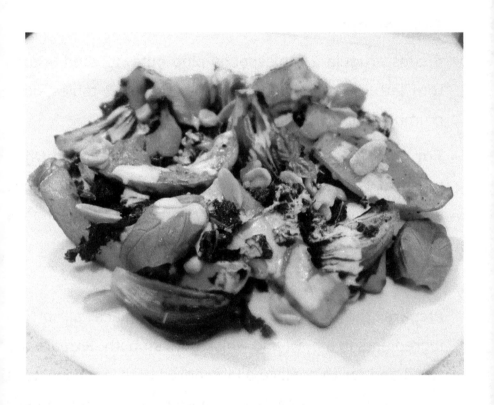

Nectarine and Arugula Salad

Preparation time: 5 minutes Cooking time: 15 minutes Servings: 8

Ingredients:

4 cups arugula 2 tablespoons pine nuts, toasted 4 cups torn lettuce 3 medium nectarines, sliced 2 tablespoons crumbled blue cheese

For the Dressing: 1/8 teaspoon salt 1 teaspoon Dijon mustard 1/8 teaspoon ground black pepper 2 teaspoons sugar 2 tablespoons raspberry vinegar 3 tablespoons olive oil

Directions:

Prepare the dressing and for this, place all of its ingredients in a bowl and whisk until smooth. Prepare the salad and for this, place all its ingredients in a bowl, toss until mixed, then drizzle with prepared dressing and stir until combined. Serve straight away.

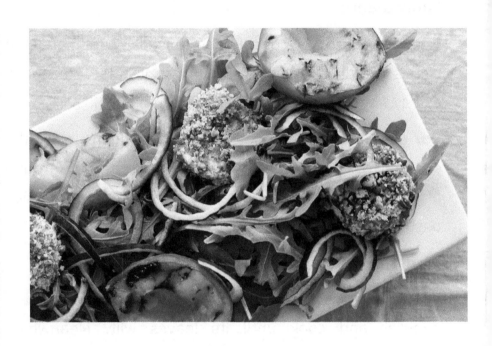

Farro, Cannellini Bean, and Pesto Salad

Preparation time: 10 minutes Cooking time: 15 minutes Servings: 4

Ingredients:

For the Pesto: 1/2 of a lemon, juiced 2 cups parsley 4 cloves of garlic, peeled 1/3 cup brazil nuts 1 teaspoon salt 1/4 cup nutritional yeast 1/2 cup olive oil

For the Salad: 19 ounces white kidney beans, cooked 2 cups farro, cooked 2 cups spinach ¼ teaspoon ground black pepper ¼ teaspoon salt 1/3 cup prepared parsley pesto ½ of a lemon, juiced

Directions:

Cook the farro until tender, add spinach in the last 5 minutes and cook until its leaves wilt. Meanwhile, prepare the pesto, and for this, place all of its ingredients in a blender and pulse until smooth. Transfer farro and spinach in a bowl, let it cool for 15 minutes, then add remaining ingredients for the salad, drizzle with pesto and toss until combined. Serve straight away.

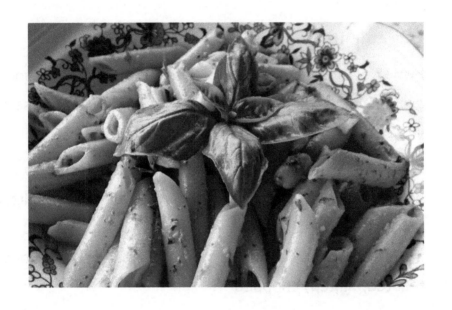

Chickpea and Kale Salad

Preparation time: 15 minutes Cooking time: 0 minute
Servings: 4

Ingredients:

For the Dressing: 2 tablespoons olive oil ½ teaspoon
ground black pepper 1 teaspoon salt 1/4 cup balsamic
vinegar 2 tablespoons maple syrup

For the Salad: 30 ounces cooked chickpeas 1 1/2 bunch
of kale, chopped 1 medium avocado, peeled, pitted,
cubed 1/2 cup dried cranberries 1/2 teaspoon salt 1 cup
diced red onion 1/2 cup chopped basil 1/2 cup almonds,
roasted, salted, chopped

Directions:

Prepare the dressing and for this, place all of its
ingredients in a bowl and whisk until smooth. Place kale
in a bowl, season with ¼ teaspoon salt, massage it into
the kale for 1 minute until soften and set aside until.
Place remaining ingredients in another bowl, toss until
combined, then top the mixture over kale and drizzle with
the dressing. Top the salad with additional almonds and
serve.

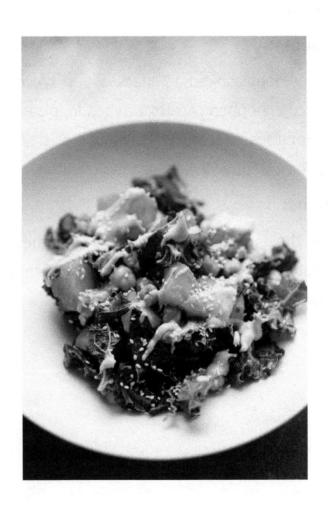

Simple Quinoa Salad

Preparation time: 10 minutes Cooking time: 0 minute Servings: 4

Ingredients:

1/2 cup quinoa, cooked 12 black olives 1/4 cup cooked corn 1/4 cup chopped carrots 1 avocado, pitted, sliced 12 cherry tomatoes, halved 1/3 teaspoon salt 1/3 teaspoon ground black pepper 2 tablespoons olive oil

Directions:

Place all the ingredients in a bowl, and then stir until incorporated. Taste the salad to adjust seasoning and serve straight away.

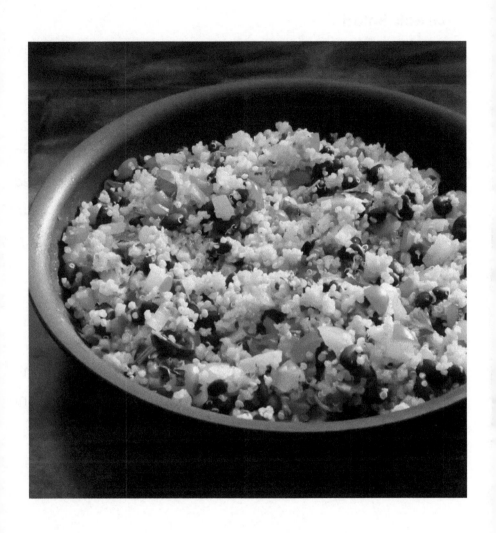

Greek Salad

Preparation time: 10 minutes Cooking time: 0 minute Servings: 4

Ingredients:

40 black olives, pitted ½ of medium red onion, peeled, sliced 4 tomatoes, sliced 1 medium cucumber, peeled, sliced 1 medium green bell pepper, cored, sliced ¼ cup tofu Feta cheese 1 tablespoon chopped oregano 1/3 teaspoon ground black pepper 1/3 teaspoon salt 2 tablespoons olive oil

Directions:

Place all the ingredients in a bowl, and then stir until incorporated. Taste the salad to adjust seasoning and serve straight away.

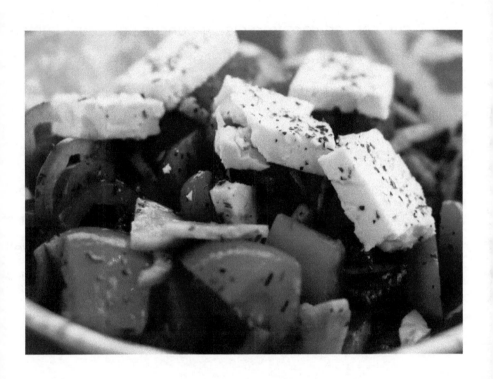

Potato Salad with Vegan Ranch Dressing

Preparation time:2 hours and 10 minutes Cooking time:0 minute Servings: 2

Ingredients:

1/2 cup cooked corn kernels 14 ounces potatoes, peeled, steamed 12 green olives ½ of medium white onion, peeled, sliced 12 cherry tomatoes, halved Vegan Ranch Dressing as needed

Directions:

Boil potatoes for 20 minutes until softened, then let cool for 10 minutes and dice them. Place diced potatoes in a bowl along with remaining ingredients and toss until well combined. Let the salad refrigerate f0r a minimum of 2 hours and then serve.

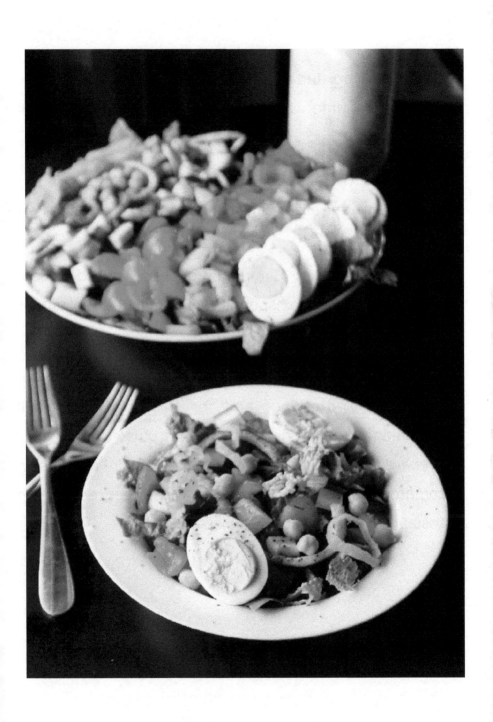

41

Zucchini Noodles with Avocado Sauce

Preparation time: 10 minutes Cooking time: 0 minute Servings: 2

Ingredients:

1 zucchini, spiralized into noodles 12 slices of cherry tomatoes

For the Dressing: 1 medium avocado, pitted, sliced 1 1/4 cup basil 2 tablespoons lemon juice 4 tablespoons pine nuts 1/3 cup water

Directions:

Prepare the dressing, and for this, place all of its ingredients in a food processor and pulse until smooth. Prepare the salad and for this, place zucchini noodles and tomato in a salad bowl, drizzle with the dressing, and toss until well coated. Serve straight away.

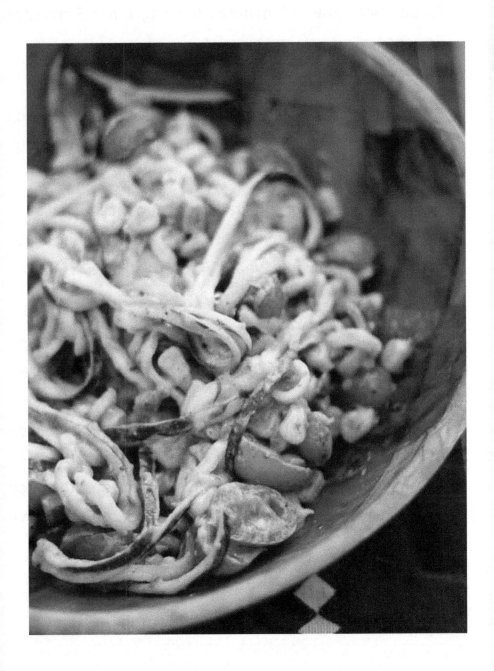

Roasted Rhubarb Salad

Preparation time: 10 minutes Cooking time: 5 minutes
Servings: 4

Ingredients:

8 cups mixed baby greens 2 cups chopped rhubarb ¼ cup
chopped walnuts, toasted 2 tablespoons sugar ½ cup
crumbled vegan goat cheese ¼ cup raisins

For the Dressing: 1 tablespoon minced shallot 2
tablespoons balsamic vinegar ¼ teaspoon ground black
pepper 1 tablespoon olive oil ¼ teaspoon salt

Directions:

Place rhubarb in a bowl, sprinkle with sugar, let them
stand for 10 minutes, then spread them in an even layer
and bake for 5 minutes at 450 degrees F until softened.
Meanwhile, prepare the dressing and for this, place all of
its ingredients in a bowl and whisk until smooth. Then
add mixed greens, toss until well coated, and then top
with roasted rhubarb, nuts, raisins, and cheese. Serve
straight away.

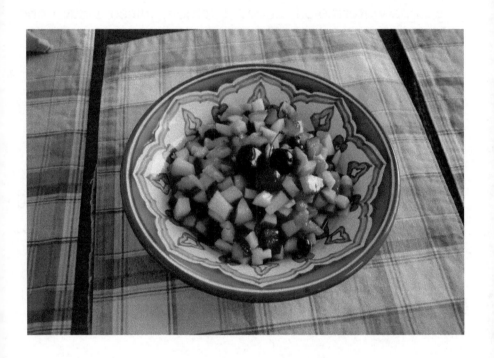

Watermelon and Mint Salad

Preparation time: 5 minutes Cooking time: 0 minute Servings: 4

Ingredients:

5 cups watermelon, cubed 1 lemon, juiced 1 cucumber, deseeded, chopped ½ teaspoon ground black pepper 1 cup mint , chopped 1 tablespoon maple syrup 2 tablespoons olive oil

Directions:

Take a large bowl and place cucumber and watermelon in it. Whisk together lemon juice, oil, and maple syrup until combined and then drizzle it over salad. Sprinkle mint on top, toss until just mixed and serve.

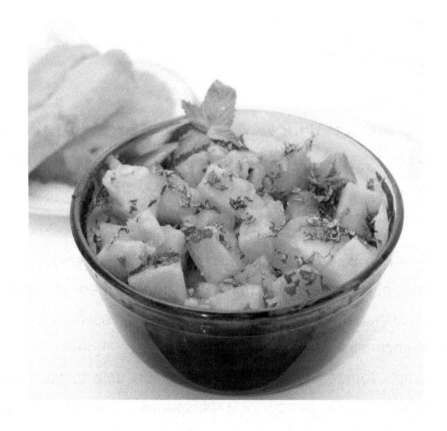

Summer Pesto Pasta

Preparation time: 10 minutes Cooking time: 10 minutes

Servings: 4

Ingredients:

For the dressing: ½ of a lemon, juiced, zested 1/2 cup basil pesto ½ teaspoon salt ½ teaspoon ground black pepper

For the Salad: 2 ears of corn, shucked 1 small green bell pepper, cored, cut into sixths 1 medium yellow squash, peeled, ½-inch sliced 1 medium zucchini, peeled, ½-inch sliced 4 green onions, trimmed, chopped 2 cups grape tomatoes, halved ½ teaspoon salt ½ teaspoon ground black pepper 2 tablespoons olive oil 1/4 cup parsley, chopped 1 pound spaghetti, whole-grain, cooked

Directions:

Prepare the dressing, and for this, place all of its ingredients in a bowl, whisk until combined, and set aside until required. Take a large bowl, place corn in it, add green onion, zucchini, squash and bell pepper, season with salt and black pepper, drizzle with oil and toss until well coated. Grill the onions for 2 minutes, grill the zucchini, squash, and bell pepper for 6 minutes until lightly charred and tender and frill the corn for 10 minutes until lightly charred, turning halfway. Cut kernels from the bowl, chop the grilled vegetables, add them to a bowl and then add remaining ingredients for the salad. Drizzle salad with prepared dressing, toss until well combined, and then serve straight away.

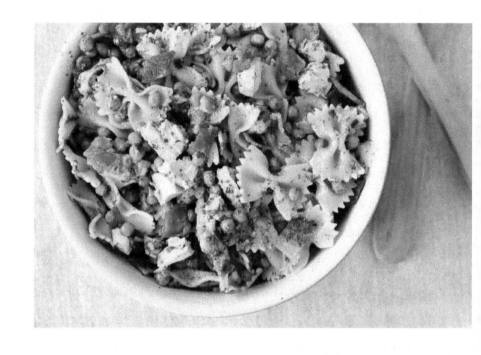

Spiralized Zucchini and Carrot Salad

Preparation time: 10 minutes Cooking time: 0 minute Servings: 6

Ingredients:

For the Salad: 2 scallions, sliced 2 large zucchini. spiralized 1 red chile, sliced 1 large carrot, spiralized

For the Dressing: 1 1/2 teaspoon grated ginger 2 teaspoons brown sugar 1/4 cup lime juice 1 tablespoon soy sauce 2 tablespoons toasted peanut oil

For Toppings: 1/2 cup chopped peanuts, roasted 1/3 cup chopped cilantro

Directions:

Prepare the dressing and for this, place all of its ingredients in a bowl and whisk until combined. Take a large bowl, place all the ingredients for the salad in it, stir until mixed, then drizzle with the dressing and toss until coated. Top the salad with nuts and cilantro and then serve straight away.

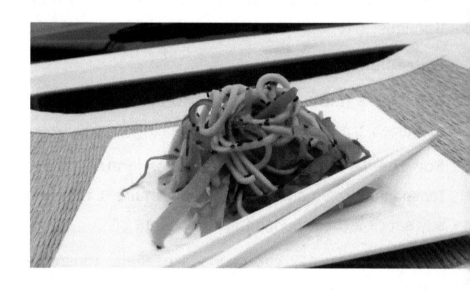

Tropical Radicchio Slaw

Preparation time: 15 minutes Cooking time: 8 minutes Servings: 6

Ingredients:

2 medium heads of radicchio, quartered 1/4 cup chopped basil leaves 2 cups chopped pineapple 1/2 teaspoon ground black pepper 1/2 teaspoon salt 2 tablespoons olive oil 2 tablespoons orange juice

Directions:

Brush radicchio with oil on both sides and then grill for 8 minutes until tender, turning halfway. When grilled, let radicchio cool for 10 minutes, then slice them thinly and place them in a bowl. Add remaining ingredients, toss until combined, and serve.

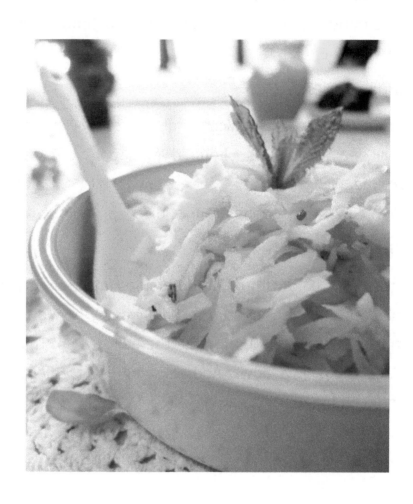

Carrot Salad with Quinoa

Preparation time: 10 minutes Cooking time: 0 minute Servings: 6

Ingredients:

For the Salad: 1 cup quinoa, cooked 3 cups grated carrots 3 scallions, sliced 2 cups sliced celery 1 bunch of cilantro, chopped ½ teaspoon minced garlic ½ teaspoon salt ½ teaspoon allspice ¼ teaspoon ground black pepper 1 tablespoon apple cider vinegar ½ teaspoon cayenne pepper ½ cup chopped almonds, toasted

For the Vinaigrette: ½ teaspoon salt 2 tablespoons honey ½ teaspoon ground black pepper ¼ cup olive oil ¼ cup apple cider vinegar

Directions: Prepare the vinaigrette and for this, place all of its ingredients in a bowl and whisk until combined. Prepare the salad and for this, place all of its ingredients in a bowl, drizzle with the vinaigrette, and toss until well combined. Serve straight away.

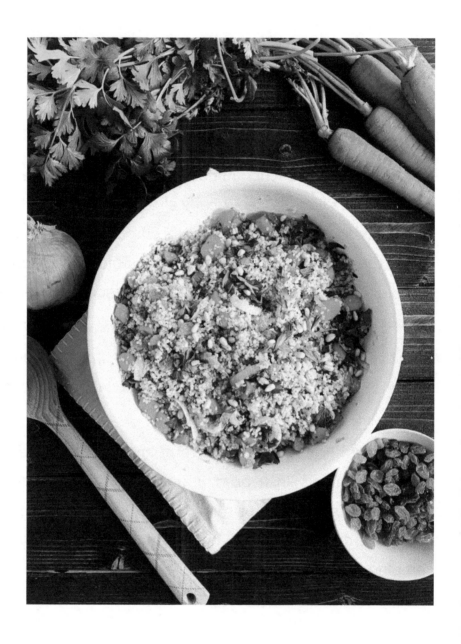

Kohlrabi Slaw

Preparation time: 10 minutes Cooking time: 0 minute Servings: 4

Ingredients:

For the Citrus Dressing: 1/2 teaspoon salt 1/4 cup honey 1 tablespoon rice wine vinegar ¼ cup of orange juice 2 tablespoons lime juice 1/4 cup olive oil

For the Salad: 6 cups kohlrabi, trimmed, peeled, cut into matchsticks ½ of a jalapeno, minced 1 orange, juiced, zested ½ cup chopped cilantro 1 lime, juiced, zested 1/4 cup chopped scallion

Directions: Prepare the dressing and for this, place all of its ingredients in a small bowl and whisk until smooth. Take a large bowl, place all the ingredients for the salad in it, top with prepared dressing and toss until well coated. Top the salad with almonds and then serve straight away.

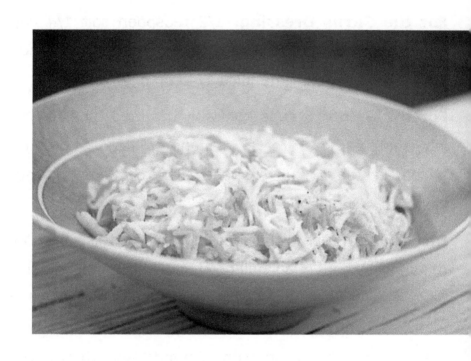

Fennel Salad with Cucumber and Dill

Preparation time: 20 minutes Cooking time: 0 minute Servings: 4

Ingredients:

2 large fennel bulbs, cored, trimmed, cored, shaved into thin slices 3 small cucumbers, shaved into thin sliced 1/2 cup chopped dill 1/4 cup sliced white onion, 1/3 teaspoon salt 1/3 teaspoon ground black pepper 1/3 cup olive oil ¼ cup lemon juice

Directions: Take a large bowl, place all the ingredients in it, and toss until well coated. Let the salad refrigerate for 15 minutes and then serve.

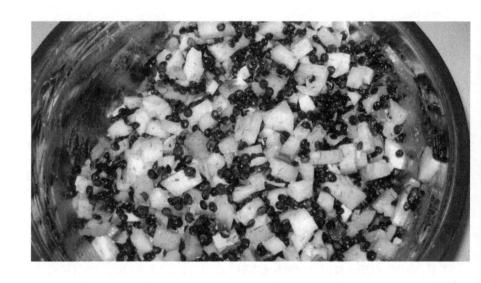

Lemon, Basil and Orzo Salad

Preparation time: 10 minutes Cooking time: 0 minute Servings: 4

Ingredients:

For the Salad: 1 cup orzo pasta, cooked 2 cups sliced cucumbers 1 cup cherry tomatoes, halved 1 cup baby arugula

For the Dressing: 2 cloves of garlic, peeled 1 lemon, zested 1 cup basil 1/3 cup olive oil ¼ teaspoon ground black pepper ½ teaspoon salt 2 tablespoons lemon juice

Directions: Prepare the dressing, and for this, place all of its ingredients in a food processor and pulse until smooth. Take a large bowl, place orzo pasta in it, add prepared dressing in it, toss until mixed, then add remaining ingredients for the salad in it and toss until just mixed. Serve straight away.

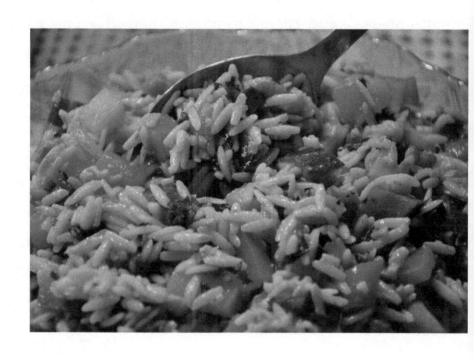

Kale Slaw

Preparation time: 10 minutes Cooking time: 0 minute Servings: 4

Ingredients:

For the Salad: ½ small head of cabbage, shredded ¼ cup mixed herbs ¼ of a medium red onion, peeled, sliced 1 small bunch of kale, cut into ribbons

For the Dressing: 1 teaspoon minced garlic ¼ teaspoon ground black pepper ¼ teaspoon salt ¼ teaspoon red chili flakes ¼ cup olive oil 1 lemon, juiced For the Topping: 1 teaspoon hemp seeds 1 teaspoon sunflower 1 teaspoon pumpkin seeds

Directions:

Prepare the dressing and for this, place all of its ingredients in a small bowl and whisk until smooth. Take a large bowl, place all the ingredients for the salad in it, top with prepared dressing and toss until well coated. Garnish the salad with all the seeds and then serve.

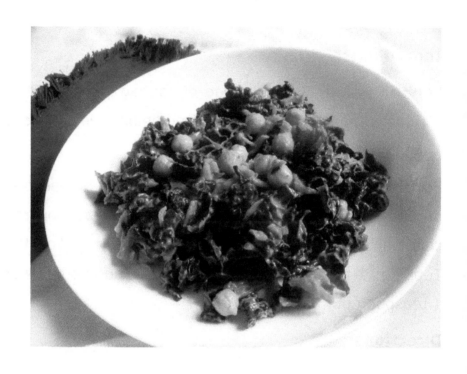

Carrot Salad with Cashews

Preparation time: 20 minutes Cooking time: 0 minute Servings: 4

Ingredients:

4 cups grated carrots 3 scallions, chopped ½ cup cilantro, chopped ½ teaspoon minced garlic 1 teaspoon minced ginger ½ teaspoon salt ¼ teaspoon cayenne pepper ¼ teaspoon ground black pepper 1 teaspoon curry powder 2 tablespoons honey ½ teaspoon ground turmeric 1/3 cup raisins ½ cup toasted cashews 1 tablespoon orange zest 3 tablespoon lime juice 1/4 cup olive oil

Directions: Take a large bowl, place all the ingredients in it, and toss until well coated. Let the salad refrigerate for 15 minutes and then serve.

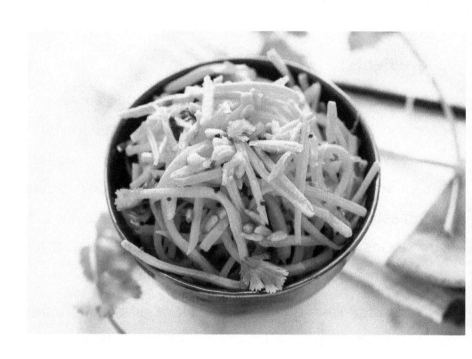

Butternut Squash Soup

Preparation Time: 15 minutes Cooking Time: 25 minutes
Servings: 6

Ingredients:

2 tbsp. olive oil 1 cup onion, chopped 1 cup cilantro 1 ginger, sliced thinly 2 cups pears, chopped ½ tsp. ground coriander Salt to taste 2 ½ lb. butternut squash, cubed 1 tsp. lime zest 26 oz. coconut milk 1 tbsp. lime juice ½ cup plain yogurt

Directions: Pour the oil into a pan over medium heat. Add the onion, cilantro, ginger, pears, coriander and salt. Stir and cook for 5 minutes. Transfer to a pressure cooker. Stir in the squash and lime zest. Pour in the coconut milk. Cook on high for 20 minutes. Release pressure naturally. Stir in the lime juice. Transfer to a blender. Pulse until smooth. Reheat and stir in yogurt before serving.

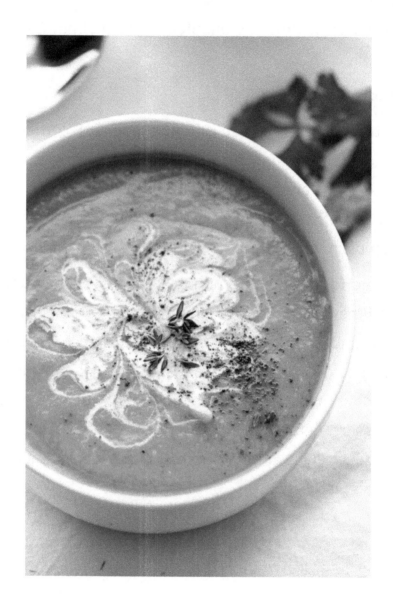

Tomato Soup with Kale & White Beans

Preparation Time: 5 minutes Cooking Time: 7 minutes Servings: 4

Ingredients:

28 oz. tomato soup 1 tbsp. olive oil 3 cups kale, chopped 14 oz. cannellini beans, rinsed and drained 1 tsp. garlic, crushed and minced ¼ cup Parmesan cheese, grated

Directions:

Pour the soup into a pan over medium heat. Add the oil and cook the kale for 2 minutes. Stir in the beans and garlic. Simmer for 5 minutes. Sprinkle with Parmesan cheese before serving.

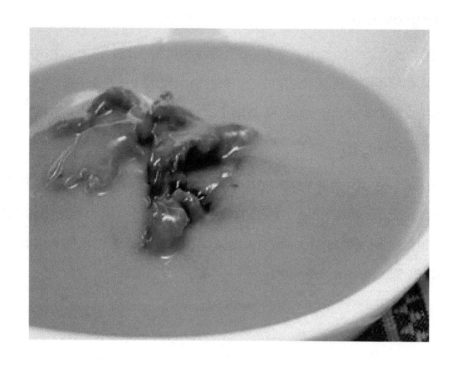

Yummy Lentil Rice Soup

Servings: 6 Preparation time: 4 hours and 15 minutes

Ingredients:

2 cups of brown rice, uncooke d 2 cups of lentils, uncooked 1/2 cup of chopped celery 1 cup of chopped carrots 1 cup of sliced mushrooms 1/2 of a medium-sized white onion, peeled and chopped 1 teaspoon of minced garlic 1 tablespoon of salt 1/2 teaspoon of ground black pepper 1 cup of vegetable broth 8 cups of water

Directions:

Using a 6-quarts slow cooker, place all the ingredients except for mushrooms and stir until it mixes properly. Cover with lid, plug in the slow cooker and let it cook for 3 to 4 hours at the high setting or until it is cooked thoroughly. Pour in the mushrooms, stir and continue cooking for 1 hour at the low heat setting or until it is done. Serve right away.

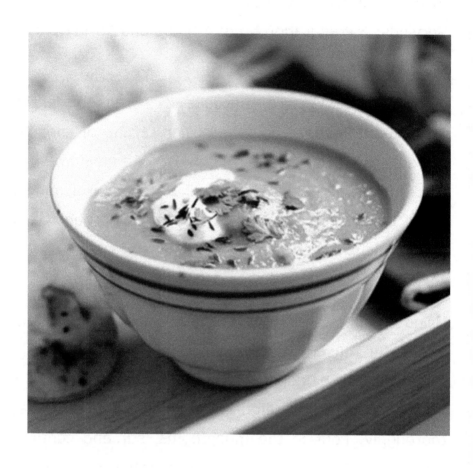

Black Bean & Corn Salad with Avocado

Total Preparation & Cooking time: 20 mins. Servings: 6

Ingredients:

1 and 1/2 cups corn kernels, cooked & frozen or canned

1/2 cup olive oil

1 minced clove garlic

1/3 cup lime juice, fresh

1 avocado (peeled, pitted & diced)

1/8 tsp. cayenne pepper

2 cans black beans, (approximately 15 oz.)

6 thinly sliced green onions

1/2 cup chopped cilantro, fresh

2 chopped tomatoes

1 chopped red bell pepper Chili powder 1/2 tsp. salt

Directions:

In a small jar, place the olive oil, lime juice, garlic, cayenne, and salt. Cover with lid; shake until all the ingredients under the jar are mixed well. Toss the green onions, corn, beans, bell pepper, avocado, tomatoes, and cilantro together in a large bowl or plastic container with a cover. Shake the lime dressing for a second time and transfer it over the salad ingredients. Stir salad to coat the beans and vegetables with the dressing; cover & refrigerate. To blend the flavors completely, let this sit a moment or two. Remove the container from the refrigerator from time to time; turn upside down & back gently a couple of times to reorganize the dressing.

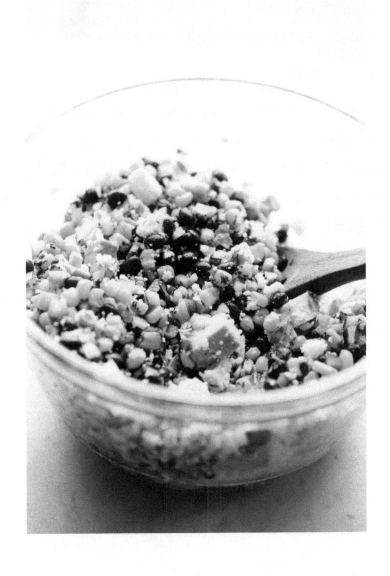

Edamame Salad

Serves: 1 Preparation Time: 15 Minutes

Ingredients:

¼ Cup Red Onion, Chopped 1 Cup Corn Kernels, Fresh 1 Cup Edamame Beans, Shelled & Thawed 1 Red Bell Pepper, Chopped 2-3 Tablespoons Lime Juice, Fresh 5-6 Basil Leaves, Fresh & Sliced 5-6 Mint Leaves, Fresh & Sliced Sea Salt & Black Pepper to Taste

Directions:

Place everything into a Mason jar, and then seal the jar tightly. Shake well before serving.

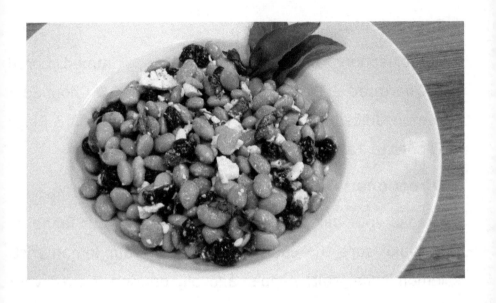

Olive & Fennel Salad

Serves: 3 Preparation Time: 5 Minutes

Ingredients:

6 Tablespoons Olive Oil 3 Fennel Bulbs, Trimmed, Cored & Quartered 2 Tablespoons Parsley, Fresh & Chopped 1 Lemon, Juiced & Zested 12 Black Olives Sea Salt & Black Pepper to Taste

Directions:

Grease your baking dish, and then place your fennel in it. Make sure the cut side is up. Mix your lemon zest, lemon juice, salt, pepper and oil, pouring it over your fennel. Sprinkle your olives over it, and bake at 400. Serve with parsley.

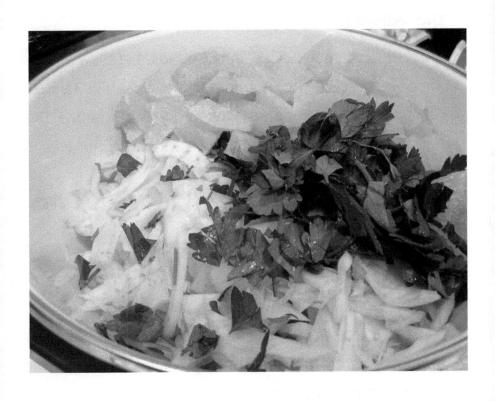

Zucchini & Lemon Salad

Serves: 2 Preparation Time: 3 Hours 10 Minutes

Ingredients:

1 Green Zucchini, Sliced into Rounds 1 Yellow Squash, Zucchini, Sliced into Rounds 1 Clove Garlic, Peeled & Chopped 2 Tablespoons Olive Oil 2 Tablespoons Basil, Fresh 1 Lemon, Juiced & Zested ¼ Cup Coconut Milk Sea Salt & Black Pepper to Taste

Directions:

Refrigerate all ingredients for three hours before serving. Interesting Facts: Lemons are popularly known as harboring loads of Vitamin C, but are also excellent sources of folate, fiber, and antioxidants. Bonus: Helps lower cholesterol. Double Bonus: Reduces risk of cancer and high blood pressure.

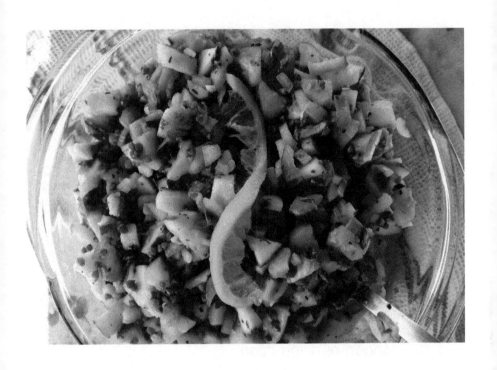

Hearty Vegetarian Lasagna Soup

Servings: 10 Preparation time: 7 hours and 20 minutes

Ingredients:

12 ounces of lasagna noodles

4 cups of spinach leaves

2 cups of brown mushrooms, sliced

2 medium-sized zucchinis, stemmed and sliced

28 ounce of crushed tomatoes

1 medium-sized white onion, peeled and diced

2 teaspoon of minced garlic

1 tablespoon of dried basil

2 bay leaves

2 teaspoons of salt

1/8 teaspoon of red pepper flakes

2 teaspoons of ground black pepper

2 teaspoons of dried oregano

15-ounce of tomato sauce

6 cups of vegetable broth

Directions:

Grease a 6-quarts slow cooker and place all the ingredients in it except for the lasagna and spinach. Cover the top, plug in the slow cooker; adjust the cooking time to 7 hours and let it cook on the low heat setting or until it is properly done. In the meantime, cook the lasagna noodles in the boiling water for 7 to 10 minutes or until it gets soft. Then drain and set it aside until the slow cooker is done cooking. When it is done, add the lasagna noodles into the soup along with the spinach and continue cooking for 10 to 15 minutes or until the spinach leaves wilts. Using a ladle, serving it in a bowl.

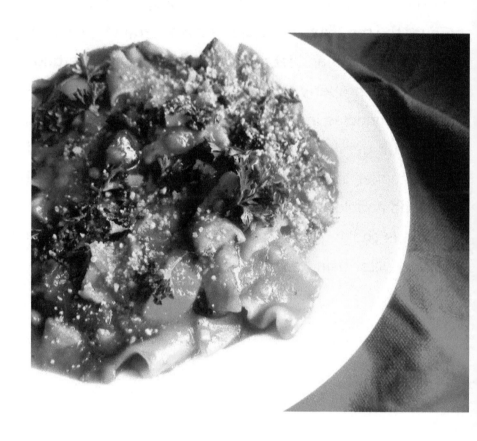

Spicy mustard

Preparation Time: 20minutes

Ingredients:

1 teaspoon of red wine vinegar ¼ teaspoon of cayenne pepper ⅛ teaspoon of chili powder

Directions: Mix and mix all INGREDIENTS in a small bowl. Save up to 1 week (maybe more time, but I haven't tried it). Try adding more INGREDIENTS to your liking

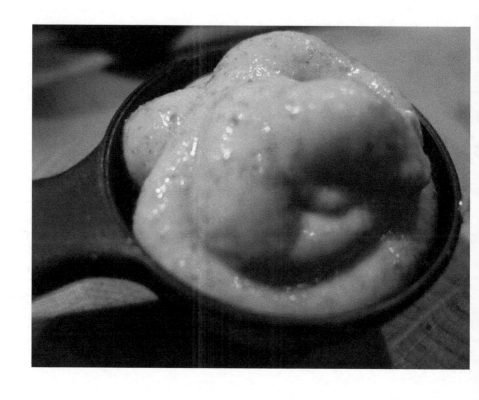

Lemon Mustard Baby Veggies

Preparation Time: 15 minutes Cooking Time: 10 minutes
Servings: 8

Ingredients:

1 clove garlic, minced 2 tablespoons fresh lemon juice 1
teaspoon Dijon mustard 2 tablespoons olive oil, divided
2 tablespoons water ½ teaspoon lemon zest 2 teaspoons
fresh basil, chopped 1 lb. baby zucchini ½ lb. baby
carrots ½ lb. baby potatoes 12 cherry tomatoes

Directions:

Mix garlic, lemon juice, mustard, half of olive oil, water
and lemon zest in a bowl. Transfer to a glass jar with lid.
Pour remaining olive oil in a pan over medium heat. Once
hot, add the vegetables. Cook until tender. Drain and
transfer in a food container. When ready to eat, reheat
veggies and toss in the lemon mustard sauce.

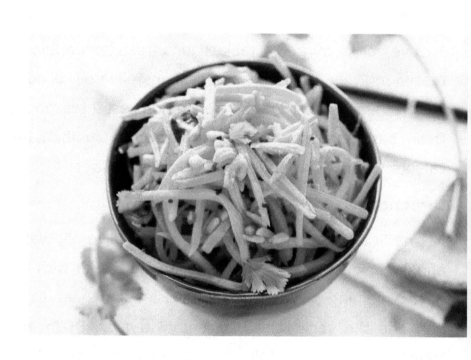

Roasted Root Vegetables

Preparation Time: 20 minutes Cooking Time: 1 hour and 10 minutes Servings: 8

Ingredients:

2 cups celery root, sliced 1 ½ cups baby carrots, peeled 8 oz. baby potatoes, sliced in half 3 parsnips, sliced 1 fennel bulb, cored and quartered 2 shallots, sliced 2 tablespoons olive oil Salt and pepper to taste

Directions:

Preheat your oven to 325 degrees F. In a baking pan, put all the root vegetables and toss to combine. Drizzle with oil and season with salt and pepper. Mix well. Bake for 1 hour. Increase temperature of your oven to 425 degrees F. Bake for 10 minutes. Transfer to a food container. Reheat in pan without oil before serving.

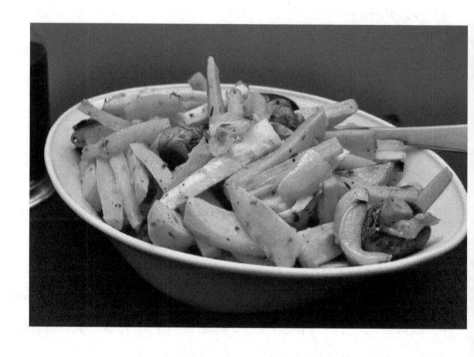

Broccoli & Cauliflower in Lemon-Dill Sauce

Preparation Time: 10 minutes Cooking Time: 20 minutes Servings: 4

Ingredients:

1 tablespoon olive oil 2 teaspoons lemon juice ½ teaspoon dried dill weed 1 clove garlic, minced Salt and pepper to taste ⅛ teaspoon dry mustard 2 cups cauliflower florets 2 cups broccoli florets Fresh dill sprigs

Directions:

Preheat your oven to 375 degrees F. Add olive oil, lemon juice, dill, garlic, salt, pepper and mustard in a glass jar with lid. Shake to blend well. In a baking pan, toss cauliflower and broccoli in 3 tablespoons lemon dill sauce. Bake in the oven for 20 minutes or until tender. Toss in the remaining sauce before serving.

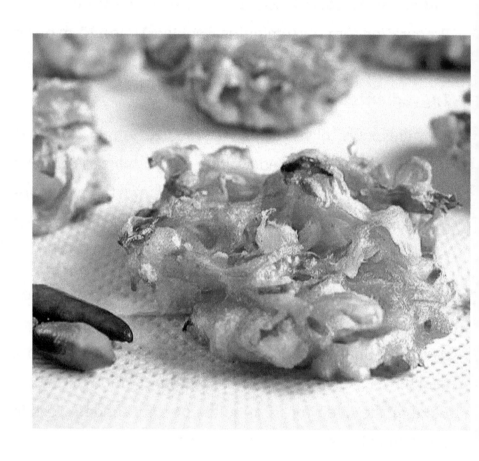

Sun-drenched tomato

Preparation Time: 30minutes

Ingredients:

1 cup raw yarn 1 cup sun-dried tomatoes (not oil-packed!) 1/2 cup water 2 garlic cloves 2 green onions 4-5 large fresh basil leaves Juice of 1/2 lemon 1/2 tsp salt Pepper pepper

Directions:

Soak the cucumber and sun-dried tomatoes in hot water for 30 minutes. Rinse and rinse. Place the licorice and sun-dried tomatoes in a food processor that fits into the S blade. Start the puree, then pour 1/2 cup into the water. Pour the puree over the sides of the bowl until smooth. Add remaining INGREDIENTS and puree until smooth. Get into the fridge.

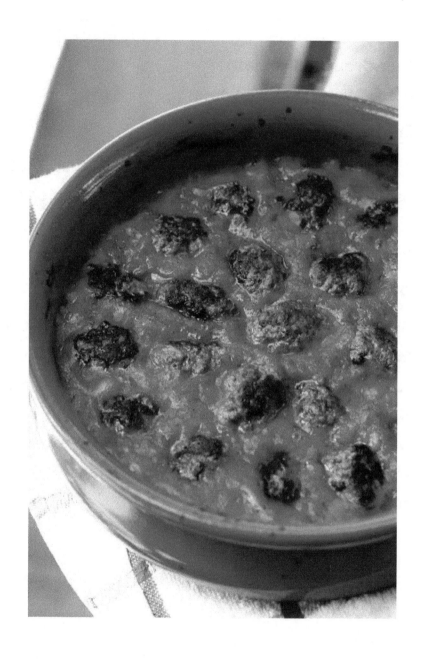

Spicy marinara sauce

Preparation Time: 30minutes

Ingredients:

1/2 sweet onion (dough) 1/4 cup vegetable broth (or water) (extra 1-2 tbsp, if needed) 3 garlic cloves (minced) 1 4-1 2 tsp crushed red pepper flakes 28 ounces canned crushed tomatoes 1/2 tsp salt (or to taste) 2 tsp dried basil 1 tsp dried oregano 1 teaspoon balsamic vinegar

Directions:

Dried onions in vegetable broth (or water) for 4-5 minutes until softened. If the onion starts to stick, add an additional 1-2 tbsp vegetable broth (or water). Add grated garlic and red pepper flakes and sauce for 1 minute. Using a blender, blend the sauce until smooth (or desired consistency). Alternatively, you can carefully slice the sauce into a blender, puree. Taste and adjust seasoning as needed. Enjoy.

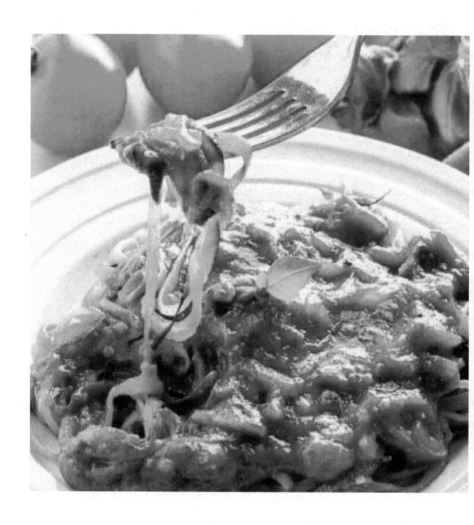

Maple Walnut Vegan Cream Cheese

Preparation Time: 30minutes

Ingredients:

1 1/2 cup raw yarn (soaked in water for several hours or overnight) 1/4 cup dairy free plain yogurt (I used tasty coconut downstairs) 4 tbsp pure maple syrup 2 tbsp fresh lemon juice 1/2 tsp salt (I used Himalayan pink salt) 1/4 cup finely chopped walnuts

Directions:

Make sure your kelps have been soaked in water for at least 3-4 hours or overnight. The longer the better. In a food processor bowl, clean the soaked licorice, yogurt, maple syrup, lemon juice and salt. Rinse sides as needed so that all INGREDIENTS are incorporated. Continue cleaning until the mixture is silky smooth. Transfer the mixture to a small bowl. Sprinkle with chopped walnuts. Store in refrigerator.

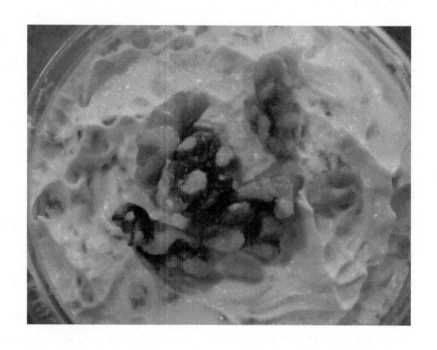

Cauliflower & Apple Salad

Serves: 4 Time: 25 Minutes Calories: 198 Protein: 7 Grams Fat: 8 Grams Carbs: 32 Grams

Ingredients:

3 Cups Cauliflower, Chopped into Florets 2 Cups Baby Kale 1 Sweet Apple, Cored & Chopped ¼ Cup Basil, Fresh & Chopped ¼ Cup Mint, Fresh & Chopped ¼ Cup Parsley, Fresh & Chopped 1/3 Cup Scallions, Sliced Thin 2 Tablespoons Yellow Raisins 1 Tablespoon Sun Dried Tomatoes, Chopped ½ Cup Miso Dressing, Optional ¼ Cup Roasted Pumpkin Seeds, Optional

Directions:

Combine everything together, tossing before serving. Interesting Facts: This vegetable is an extremely high source of vitamin A, vitamin B1, B2 and B3.

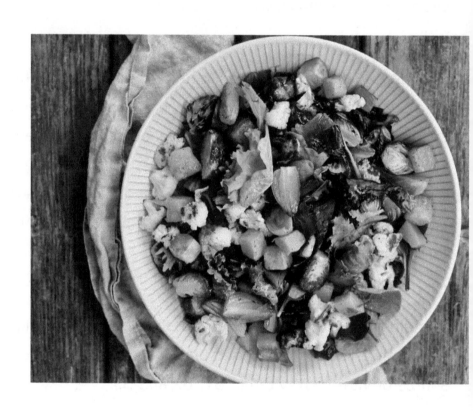

Spinach & Orange Salad

Serves: 6 Time: 15 Minutes Calories: 99 Protein: 2.5 Grams Fat: 5 Grams Carbs: 13.1 Grams

Ingredients:

¼ -1/3 Cup Vegan Dressing 3 Oranges, Medium, Peeled, Seeded & Sectioned ¾ lb. Spinach, Fresh & Torn 1 Red Onion, Medium, Sliced & Separated into Rings

Directions:

Toss everything together, and serve with dressing. Interesting Facts: Spinach is one of the most superb green veggies out there. Each serving is packed with 3 grams of protein and is a highly encouraged component of the plant-based diet.

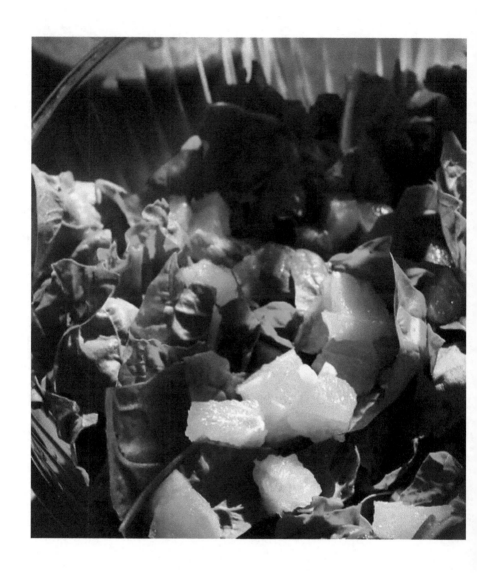

Mushroom Pasta

Preparation time: 10 minutes Cooking time: 30 minutes
Servings: 4

Ingredients:

1 Cup Coconut Milk 1 ½ Cups Mushrooms, Sliced 1
Teaspoon Arrowroot 1 Cup Pasta 2 Cups Water

Directions: Press sauté and then pour in a little bit of
your coconut milk, adding in your mushrooms. Cook for
three minutes, and then stir in your pasta, water and the
remaining milk. Secure the lid, and then cook on high
pressure for seven minutes. Use a quick release, and
then press sauté again. Whisk in our arrowroot powder,
allowing it to simmer until it thickens. Serve warm once
thickened.

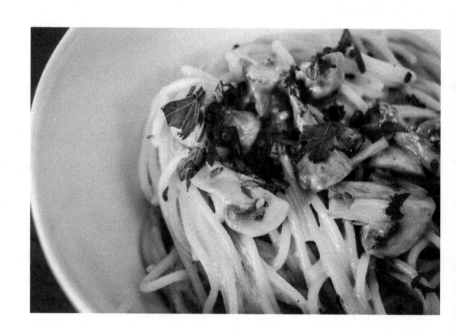

Gobi Masala

Preparation time: 10 minutes Cooking time: 30 minutes Servings: 4

Ingredients:

1 Clove Garlic, Minced 1 White Onion, Diced 1 Teaspoon Cumin Seeds 1 Tablespoons olive Oil 1 Head Cauliflower, Chopped 1 Teaspoon Cumin 1 Tablespoon Coriander ½ Teaspoon Sea Salt, Fine 1 Cup Water ½ Teaspoon Garam Masala Cooked Rice to Serve

Directions:

Put your instant pot on sauté and press low, and then add the oil in. once it's hot cook your cumin seeds for thirty seconds, and stir often to keep it from burning. Add the onion in, cooking for another three minutes. Keep stirring to keep it from burning. Add in the garlic, cooking for another half a minute. Add the coriander, cauliflower, cumin, garam masala, water and salt. Lock your lid and cook on high pressure for one minute. Use a quick release, and serve over rice.

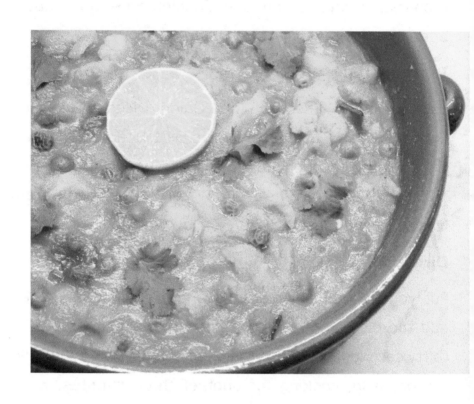

Vegan Hoppin' John

Preparation time: 10 minutes Cooking time: 30 minutes Servings: 4

Ingredients:

1 Tablespoon Olive Oil 1 Red Bell Pepper, Diced 1 Sweet Onion, Diced 2 Tomatoes, Chopped 1 Teaspoon Vegan Worcestershire Sauce 1 Teaspoon chili Powder ½ Teaspoon Thyme ½ Teaspoon Garlic Powder Sea Salt & Black Pepper to Taste 1 Cup Black Eyed Peas, Rinsed 3 ¼ Cups Vegetable Stock 1 Cup Peas, Frozen 3 Cups Kale, Fresh & Chopped 2 Cups Brown Rice, Cooked

Directions:

Press sauté and set I tot low and then add the oil. Once it's hot cook the bell pepper and onion for three minutes, stirring often. Turn off sauté and then add in the chili powder, tomatoes, vegan Worcestershire sauce, garlic powder, salt, pepper, garlic powder, black eyed peas and stock. Seal the lid, and cook on high pressure for twenty minutes. Use a natural pressure release for twenty minutes and then finish with a quick release. Add the frozen peas, kale and rice, and stir well.

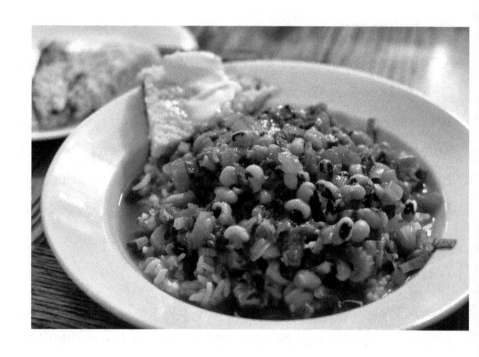

Vegan Ratatouille

Preparation time: 10 minutes Cooking time: 30 minutes Servings: 4

Ingredients:

1 Eggplant, Sliced 2 Zucchini, Sliced 1 Tablespoon Olive Oil 3 Tomatoes, Sliced 2 Cups Water

Directions:

Pour your water in, and then get out a baking dish. Layer your eggplant, tomatoes and zucchini until you run out of ingredients. Spritz with olive oil, and then add in your trivet. Put the baking dish on top of the trivet. Secure the lid, and cook on high pressure for ten minutes. Use a natural release before serving.

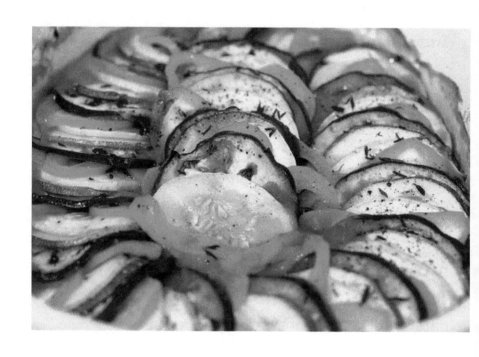

Lightning Source UK Ltd.
Milton Keynes UK
UKHW020652240521
384262UK00001B/69